Off The Mat

Off The Mat

✦

Thoughts From a Yoga Practice

Nicole DiSalvo Billa, RYT

iUniverse, Inc.
New York Lincoln Shanghai

Off The Mat
Thoughts From a Yoga Practice

iUniverse books may be ordered through booksellers or by contacting:

iUniverse
2021 Pine Lake Road, Suite 100
Lincoln, NE 68512
www.iuniverse.com
1-800-Authors (1-800-288-4677)

ISBN-13: 978-0-595-41740-7 (pbk)
ISBN-13: 978-0-595-86080-7 (ebk)
ISBN-10: 0-595-41740-X (pbk)
ISBN-10: 0-595-86080-X (ebk)

Printed in the United States of America

For Michael, Julian, and Kai—my greatest teachers

Contents

Introduction xi

Off the Mat. 1

Holding Your Tongue. 3

At the Crossroads 5

Ripping Up Rugs 7

For Mother's Day 9

Declaration of Independence. 11

New Tattoo. 13

The Ides of March. 15

The Spring of Our Content 17

Listening to the Body 19

Wrestling with time 21

It's All For the Good. 23

The Fruits of Our Labors 25

Learning to Read. 28

The Tyranny of Expectations 30

Enough is Enough. 32

Season of Wonder. 34

Meeting Resistance 36

Ebb and Flow 38

Learning to Fall 40

The Only Way Out is Through. 42

Forward bends and the art of surrender.. 44

The Eight Limbs of Yoga. 49

After Yama, Niyama 51

Ahhh, Asana 54

Breath of Life. 56

Turning Inward. 58

Unity from Diversity 60

Journey to the Center 62

Who am I?. 64

Acknowledgments

First and foremost, great thanks and appreciation to Carrie Parker Gastelu. She was my first yoga teacher, and after six years of taking her class, I am still amazed at how much she has to teach. I'd also like to offer thanks to Jillian Pransky, for her guidance during (and after!) teacher training. Great thanks as well to Sheryl Edsall; she has been a great inspiration. I offer thanks to all of my teachers and students for the light they have brought into my life.

As a writer, I was first encouraged by a teacher named Barbara Corcoran, who saw a seed of talent in me when I was a very troubled teenager. During times of hopelessness, when it seemed I wouldn't ever get on a healthy path, her words of encouragement often came back to me. At Bard College I had the privilege to study non-fiction writing under William Weaver; he was a great mentor for me during my last year at Bard. Great thanks as well to my Philosophy professors at Bard; Daniel Berthold, William Griffiths, and Bard College President Leon Botstein. Their incredible teaching sparked my interest in the 'great questions' of life that has since become a passion.

And of course thank you to the wonderful family and friends that support me, especially Mom, Granny, and Leandra. I count you all among my blessings. *Namaste.*

Introduction

Most of the following essays were written for my monthly Yoga newsletter, Off the Mat, over the past three years. I began writing these pieces as a way to share some of the ways that Yoga has changed my life for the better. Of course, I have the opportunity to do that in classes, but I can only talk for so long at the beginning of class before my students start to get antsy. The personal essay format gave me a chance to go a little deeper into some of the ways Yoga practice and philosophy relate to life off the mat.

Also included are several previously unpublished essays, as well as a series on the eight limbs of Yoga that were originally written for Devotion Yoga's *E-connection* newsletter.

Many times, when I return to a work written a year or two in the past, I feel no urge to get that writing out into the world. In preparing this book, there were a few pieces that I felt didn't stand the test of time, and so they were not included in this work. But on the whole, when I re-read these essays, I felt I could still stand behind the words I had written as long ago as three years.

I offer these essays in thanks to the practice of Yoga, and in hope that these words will prove useful to those who are reflecting on their own practice. *Namaste.*

Off the Mat

Yoga is a great inward journey. As yogis we practice *svadhyaya,* or self-study. In the beginning this may only occur on the mat, while we are practicing. Perhaps we notice jealousy of other students, or resentment of particular poses. We notice how we react to challenges, and how we react to pleasure in our practice. As we integrate our Yoga practice into our life off the mat, we begin to practice svadhyaya more often, frequently dropping back into our witness consciousness to observe our selves. The inward journey changes the way we look outward.

One of my first big Yoga 'aha' moments came after only about 4 months of practicing Yoga. At the time we lived in a small apartment in a complex of garden apartments. We had a very nasty downstairs neighbor. He complained about our dogs, he complained about our baby's rare crying, and he greeted any smile or hello with a blank stare. He was very, very proud of his car. It was a nice car, admittedly. He would purposely park the car in the street in front of our doors, which were right next to each other. He would try to take up enough space that no other cars could get in front or behind him. That really got my husband and I upset. If we couldn't park in front of the apartment, we would have to go around the back to the parking lot, which was a pretty long walk when you're carrying a baby and a few bags of groceries or laundry. One day my husband decided to force the issue. There was just enough space for him to park behind our neighbor's car, if he bumped our neighbor's bumper. So he did it. Our neighbor must have been watching from his window, and he came out screaming. His anger, rage, and hate poured out, all over a tapped bumper. My husband, who is about as even-tempered a guy as you can get, had had it and was not about to take the rage sitting down, and started shouting back.

Upstairs I felt my blood begin to boil. My heart started to pound and I grabbed the baby, ready to join the fray. I couldn't wait to unleash the bad feelings of the last year on our neighbor. Halfway down the stairs something happened. I took a breath. Something big happened, and so quickly. I saw my neighbor as a sad, lonely man, pathetically attached to his car. I felt his sadness; what else would compel him to react that way to a tap on his car's bumper? In that blinding instant I saw myself as well; how quick I could be to anger, how

1

self-righteous was my rage. I saw that pattern as it had been repeated through my whole life. I went downstairs and handed the baby to my husband, and sent him upstairs. I let my neighbor vent at me for a few minutes. I apologized profusely. I explained how hard it was for me when I had to park behind the building. He was mollified, and we went back to our apartments in peace. He didn't change in the time we lived there, he never became friendly, but we didn't have any other problems with him either.

It was a small incident, but it was the first time I realized how big Yoga practice really was; how it would change everything about my life, not just my body. In reality all that happened was that we avoided a scene that could have turned pretty ugly. In my mind it was huge; I had a glimpse of my patterned reactions to things, and of how just taking a breath could change those reactions. Five years from then, I still see the effects of the practice. This is how Yoga can change the world. If one person at a time, we act out of love and peace instead of anger, eventually things change. This is part of the work of the yogi; to carry out into the world the fruits of our practice.

Lokah Samasta Sukhino Bhavantu *May all beings, everywhere, be happy and free. And may the thoughts, words, and actions of my own life contribute, in some way, to that happiness and to that freedom for all.*

A stone cast into water sends ripples in all directions—Zen koan

Holding Your Tongue

Yoga has its own code of ethics, the *yamas* and *niyamas*. The first of these is *ahimsa*, translated as non-harming, or nonaggressiveness. I've written about ahimsa before, in the context of asana practice and how we must learn to listen to the body. Lately I've been thinking about, and working with, this concept again. I think *ahimsa*'s place as the first of the *yamas* is important; it is the hardest to practice, but it is the gateway that leads to all of the others.

The obvious meaning of *ahimsa* is easy to understand. Nonviolence; okay, so we're meant not to hurt each other. But Yoga takes it farther; we are also meant not to hurt or be aggressive to ourselves. This may be a bit more of a stretch, but *ahimsa* goes even further. We are meant, I think, to extend this nonaggressivenss, nonharming, to every aspect of our being.

When you start seeing ahimsa in this way, as something to practice in every interaction with the universe, there are opportunities for it in every aspect of our lives. *Ahimsa* is difficult, but it is not just work; it has the power to transform our lives in the most amazing way.

The other night my husband and I got in a little tiff. To be more accurate, I am very pregnant and not exactly hormonally balanced at the moment, and I picked a bit of a fight. Now, for the first few hours afterwards, the thought of *ahimsa* was the farthest thing from my mind. I was just waiting for him to come home from work so I could finish what I'd started. He, of course, just wanted a quiet evening at home.

Luckily something stopped me from flying off the handle. I took a moment to ask for guidance. Nothing came to mind, and when our son was finally asleep I was ready to start venting at my poor husband. But before I could start talking, I heard the word *ahimsa*. So I waited. As I lay there, I could hear the words I wanted to say echoing in my own head. I heard them as if for the first time. Everything I wanted to say was accusatory, and meant to wound.

It was a moment of clarity. For the first time I could see how all of the things I was about to say were cruel, and unnecessary. I felt as if there was a lens looking back over the past nine years of my time with my husband, and every time we had argued my words had come out of anger, rather than love. In that instant I felt my understanding completely transformed.

This is not to say that we should never express anger. But maybe it's a good idea to pause sometimes, bearing in mind the idea of *ahimsa*. Our lives are different when we pause, and question ourselves, before we speak. Ask yourself, where are these words coming from? What is the motivation?

What would the world be like if we all did this? Imagine if we took a breath before yelling at each other, every single time. Imagine if we all brought to mind the idea of *ahimsa* before we spoke. Sometimes the way to follow *ahimsa* is simply to say nothing; to hold your tongue until the words you are about to speak come from a place of love.

"We must train our sensitivity to the fact that we are not alone in the universe but are interdependent cells of a cosmic body...Even if we do not mean to harm another person, our coldness or indifference is a form of harming. Whenever we are not present as love, we inevitably reduce our own life and the life in others..."
Georg Feuerstein, from the essay "Is Nonharming (Ahimsa) an Old-fashioned Value?"

At the Crossroads

We are all the time engaged in decision-making or decision-avoidance. The more consciously we live, the more we realize that life is really an incessant stream of potential decisions.

Georg Feurstein, "Living in the Dark Age (Kali-Yuga)", in <u>The Deeper Dimension of Yoga</u>

A few weeks ago, at a friend's birthday party, I found myself in conversation with a stranger. We spoke for a few minutes of inconsequential things, but soon we got to the deep stuff. She had just turned thirty-five; she was talking of her longing for a child before it was too late. At the end of our conversation she said, "Well, now isn't a good time. I'm really in a time of transition right now, starting a new job." Then she stopped, just for a second, and said, "Really we can always change; no matter how old you are there's always another chance."

I didn't think about it much at the time; we were interrupted for cake. But her words came back to me later. So often we think of our lives as stagnant, with transformation only possible at set times and in set situations. You turn eighteen and people expect to see you change. You finish high school or college, change is expected. Only at life's passages do people expect change from us, and do we therefore expect change in ourselves.

Yoga teaches us that this isn't, in fact, the case. Transformation is always an option. In fact, it's a constant. As we practice our svadhyaya (self-study), we notice how many of our responses to stimuli are habitual. We begin to create space in our minds as well as our bodies. We find a split second between the stimulus and our reaction to it, and we can take that time to choose the reaction we will have. We can change our habitual reactions any time we become aware of them.

In my first yoga class my gut reaction was anger. The poses hurt; why was someone trying to hurt me? It was all I could do not to run out of class. As time went on I found space to notice my reactions before they took hold of me. Now when I encounter a painful posture, I can drop back into my body and listen to its cues. I can choose to react to a pose I can't do with humor and a light heart

5

instead of anger. The way I react to things is up to me; thus I can shape my own life.

We can take this decision-making off the mat, for the big things and the little things in life. When stuck in traffic, we can choose to enjoy a few minutes to think instead of reacting with impatience. And when it comes to the big things, we can remember that with every breath, we are given another chance to make a choice.

Every moment, we are at the crossroads.

Ripping Up Rugs

A few weeks ago I spent a Friday ripping up carpet. It's not the most pleasant job in the world. There's a lot of dirt underneath old wall-to-wall carpet. Along the edges of the room is tacking. Tacking is strips of wood with tacks sticking out; tacking holds the carpet down, and is glued to the floor when the carpet is installed. Ripping up the rug wasn't the hard part. That was actually kind of pleasant. The tacking was the hard part. To get it out, I had to insert a little crowbar into the tiny space between the tacking wood and the hardwood floor. Then I had to use my strength to pry up the wood, glued in place 12 years ago. Over the course of a few hours I figured out a better way. I used a hammer to get the crowbar deeper in; it was then easier to pry up the wood. I learned how to pry up staples and nails using the back of the hammer.

It wasn't the most traditionally fun way to spend Memorial Day weekend. But I felt good anyway. My muscles were sore and tired. Everything hurt. We worked all day Friday and most of Saturday. We moved furniture, cleaned and bleached the wood underneath the carpets. Physically I was beat, but mentally I felt wonderful.

'Being handy' has never been one of the ideas I held about myself. But every time I try something around the house, I'm pleasantly surprised. I've always thought I was clumsy, artsy, and impractical. That's not really true. Since we moved in with my grandmother, I've painted a door, mowed lawns, learned to garden, fixed a toilet, and ripped up a carpet. From an early age I was labeled "creative," and at the same time, "not scientific or mathematical", as if those things couldn't go together. Through Yoga I've come to love anatomy, and biology, and all sorts of things I never thought I would understand. I love reading books meant for the amateur scientist. I've discovered a passion for history.

Practicing Yoga has changed my attitude to trying new things, but the change has been so gradual I've only just realized it. In Yoga practice, we are constantly challenged. First we have stiff muscles and joints. Later, when we've loosened out bodies a little, we have the challenge of learning to focus our concentration. If we stick with the practice, we expand our limits. Every challenge we meet changes our idea of what we can and can't do.

We start out saying "I can't balance on one foot." A few months or years later, we are as stable as flamingos. We learn that we have the power to transform ourselves, and that there are very few limits to what we can do.

Think about the labels you put on yourself, especially the negative ones. Then play with the idea that all of them are wrong. Try something you never thought you could do. Surprise yourself.

We become as big as the containers we put ourselves in.

For Mother's Day

Last week I took the train from Hoboken to Fair Lawn. I sat and looked out the window. On the train I like to savor the peace and quiet. I'm not alone very often; when I am, I enjoy every second. At Secaucus loads of people boarded the train. I watched a gaggle of boys in sailor suits come on and take the few rows of seats behind me. There were five or six of them. They looked so young. At first I thought they were cadets of some kind, but from their conversation it was clear that they were soldiers. Their faces were bare, their eyes were bright, and their voices were loud. The one in charge had bright blue eyes. They were the kind of boys you'd want your daughter to bring home. I tried to go back to reading my book, but I couldn't. They were talking and I couldn't help but listen.

"Well, I heard that in Vietnam you didn't last more than 3 days if you weren't commissioned…"

"Yeah, the officers have it better, they just stay on the ship."

"We'll be there by July…"

Their conversation went in spurts. It was hard to follow. But they kept coming back to Vietnam. To how long one could have expected to have lived if one had gone there. To what kind of food one would have eaten. But the conversation stayed in the past and in the hypothetical. None of them said the word Iraq.

Before I got off the train their conversation changed. The leader, the one whose house they were going to, started talking about how it had been so long since he'd been home that he had forgotten his own phone number. It seemed he had brought home friends whose own mothers were far away. Who would pick them up? Names were rattled off, he was proud to name the people who cared for him and waited for his return. "I could call my brother, or Michael, or Paul, my mom will be home at 5…"

My stop came before theirs. For some reason I was crying. I wished I could say something to them on my way out. Be careful. Thank you for wanting to protect us. For your mother's sake, stay home.

May all be well with mankind. May the leaders of the earth protect it in every way by keeping to the right path. May there be goodness for those who know the earth to be sacred. May all the worlds be happy. May the rains fall on time and may the earth yield its produce in abundance. May this country be free of disturbance and may we be free from fear.

Ashtanga yoga closing chant.

Declaration of Independence

A few weeks ago I had a revelation. I know it's one many women have had before me, and I know we've all heard it before. It's time to stop wasting time hating my body, wishing it were thinner, or curvier, or stronger, or different in any way. I've believed this with my head. But all along I've spent time thinking about how I can trick my body into getting thinner, when my body likes the weight it's at. For years I've looked in the mirror seeing nothing but imperfection. I've sent daggers of hatred into myself. I've alternately starved and binged, and the few times I managed to get 'skinny enough' were also the lowest points in my life. My revelation happened after a lovely yoga practice; for the first time I felt with my heart and not just my head, that it was time to love my body.

After my revelation, I decided I'd had enough. I will no longer judge my body based on how it looks. I will not keep criticizing myself. I will revel in the way my body actually feels. Physically, I feel stronger and healthier than I did when I was eighteen. I can walk for miles, swim, hike, run, and do almost anything. Yoga has made me strong, limber, and agile. I feel at home in my body in a way I never did when I was busy starving it.

The more I've thought about this issue of body hatred, the more I see the way Yoga shows us a different path. The first *yama*, or ethical guideline of the yogi, is *ahimsa*, which translates roughly as non-harming. Hating your body is not *ahimsa*; every time you criticize yourself, you are hurting yourself. The self-hating thoughts do not help us in any way.

Being so focused on our external bodies, we forget the important things about our selves. Our culture values the externals, and most people don't seem very happy that way. If I use an external value system I will always find myself wanting. I am not model skinny. I am not rich. By those standards, I am not successful. So I will live my life according to different standards. My Yoga practice reminds me that my emotional and spiritual well-being are as important as the physical.

So I'm declaring myself independent. My only goal with my weight is that it will be a healthy one. I will no longer compare myself to women on television or magazines. I will not look in the mirror and hate my hips. I will love my potbelly even though fat tummies are 'unattractive'. (After all, my son likes to lay his head on it; it's nice and soft.) I will remember that the important things really are inside. I'm going spend a few minutes every day feeling lucky that I have enough to eat and a whole and healthy body.

New Tattoo

Most of you know my old tattoo. It was an ugly, mean-looking snake. When it was originally done, I hated the bottom, so after a few months I got that covered up with a design that I really didn't like very much. At first I liked that tattoo. I got it when I was 19, and had just finished my first year of college. I thought I was making a statement. I meant it as a rejection of the traditional idea that the snake is evil. The snake in many cultures is a symbol of wisdom, and I desperately needed some of that. Plus the snake is ever changing, growing and molting and regrowing a new skin. Another idea I could get into.

Unfortunately, the reality didn't match my ideals. With the design at the bottom, the tattoo looked like a scorpion. And it was ugly. Instead of a wise, sublime creature, my snake was mean looking. Within a few years I came to hate the snake on my arm. I tried not to look at it, ever. I hated seeing my reflection when I wore sleeveless shirts. It looked hard, a little masculine, tough. It meant something to me in a symbolic way; it was gotten as I was coming out of a dark place and getting it was a mark of that passage. But as I got older and made peace with my life the more uncomfortable I felt with my ugly tattoo. It was a mark of rebellion and I was no longer rebelling. It was a sign of anger and I wasn't quite so angry anymore. I hated when people asked about it, and I hated my reaction more. With every, "Is that a scorpion? What is that thing?" I reacted defensively. I could feel myself shutting down, rage and resentment filling me. I always wanted to scream, "I hate this thing. I got it when I was young and stupid; can we pretend it's not there? Please!"

So yesterday I covered up the old tattoo. It's always a journey, marking your body. Sitting for two hours in pretty serious pain gives you cause to think about things. My wonderful tattoo artist drew on my ugly tattoo with a regular ballpoint pen. Before my eyes I saw a flower grow where the design had been. Vines sprung up around it, and a vine with little leaves covered what used to be the snake. Over two hours he made what was ugly become beautiful.

The process made me think of the ways Yoga, and contemplative practice, has made so much of what was ugly in my life become beautiful. On Friday my car died, and a new battery cost me $100. Coincidentally, I had just deposited an extra $100 I had made in the bank. In the old days, I would have been so angry. "Isn't that the way it always is? You get extra and it gets taken away…" But instead the experience cheered up my whole evening. I had spent the day driving with Julian, but when the car died he was safely at home. The car stopped working literally 200 feet from my mechanic's garage. It was five o'clock on Friday, and they were just closing up, but they happened to have the right battery in stock, and fixed it before they left. And the $100? Thank god I had put in that extra money.

And now when I look back at the past, I find it easier and easier all the time to see the beauty that went with the bad parts, and how the suffering changed my life for the better.

On the way home from the tattoo shop, Julian couldn't stop looking at the new tattoo. "The ugly snake is gone—it's hiding in the vine!" he said. And he's right. It's gone, but it's also still there. You can make out the shape of it if you know what you're looking for. But it's been turned into something beautiful.

"Consider the possibility that you may be believing untruths about yourself, convictions that are causing you and others to suffer needlessly, and then consciously go inward and *experience* yourself. Allow yourself to experience the truth of your reality—your inherent creative goodness, and acknowledge your right to know the truth about yourself. And if doing that makes you feel absolutely fabulous for no apparent reason, then so be it." Erich Schiffman, in <u>Yoga: The Spirit and Practice of Moving Into Stillness</u>

The Ides of March

I think this is the hardest time of the year. For almost six months the world around us has been cold. Winter is the season of rest and hibernation, of retrenching. This is a wonderful part of the cycle of our being, but I think I've had enough. We've had a few nice days here and there, just enough to tease us with the coming of spring. Underneath the snow the world is ready to burst back into life. Even though it's cold, the days have been getting longer. Some of my bulbs, confused by the warm weather a few weeks ago, have already sent stems and leaves to be frozen above the surface. As I wait for the world to warm up, the snow falls outside.

Last Friday I listened to the weather report. I heard the first news of the storm we're dealing with now. Then I heard of below-average temperatures for the next week. My spirits crashed, and I actually got angry. Until that moment I hadn't realized how long I had been waiting for spring. Through yoga practice I've definitely gotten better at living in the present moment. All winter I've tried to accept the season for what it was. When people complained about the dark, and the cold, the snow and the wind, I tried to keep silent. I spent my outdoor walks appreciating the strange beauty that is winter. But I guess I've run out of patience.

For months now I've been waiting for spring, and waiting for my new baby. I know spring will come; the wait for spring is one filled with the most delicious anticipation. It's inevitable; you can't stop the spring from coming. I know the baby will come too; that wait, though, I'm having a little more trouble with. Ever since we had a false alarm test result, I've been a nervous wreck. The whole tenor of my 'wait' for the baby has changed. Just as earlier in winter I wasn't waiting for spring but enjoying winter, before the test I wasn't waiting for the baby but enjoying my pregnancy. Now, at the end of winter, I am simply waiting for spring, and instead of enjoying my pregnancy I am simply waiting for the baby. My fears and anxieties have taken away all my patience; now I feel like I'm waiting, in fear, with bated breath.

Yoga practice has calmed me; in the midst of worry, I can remember that I am not in control. This would seem to be scary, but in fact it's very reassuring. I have no control over the outcome of what I'm worried about. I have no way to know the baby will be fine until I hold him in my arms. Remembering that makes the next breath come easier. In times of stress, I try always to go back to the wisdom I have gotten from Yoga practice, which I have seen proven in my life again and again. Whatever comes into my life is exactly what I need to learn. As long as I stick to the practice of Yoga, I will be able to remember that and be able to keep things in perspective.

Faith is the important thing, whatever it is you have faith in.

'Everything
Changes in this world
*   But flowers will open*
Each spring
Just as usual.'   Zen folk saying

The Spring of Our Content

As winter finally draws to a close, I have been thinking a lot about the energetic changes that come with the seasons. We are moving from a time of turning inward to a time of blossoming out. Thinking about what winter means has brought me to the idea of *svadhyaya,* Sanskrit for self-study.

Svadhyaya is one of the three ways to find the state of Yoga, according to Patanjali's <u>Yoga Sutras.</u> It is an idea that also turns up in modern thought. The basis of psychoanalysis is Sigmund Freud's exhortation to make the unconscious conscious. Through self-observation, we come to know ourselves. We find the thoughts and feelings that lie behind our actions; we start to see our motivators. It is this process that allows us to change and to grow.

Yet *svadhyaya* is not a process that makes us into instantly happy people. While we are gathering information about ourselves, we may turn up some things that are not so savory.

In the first six months of my Yoga practice, with *svadhyaya,* I learned quite a few things about myself. I learned that I was preoccupied with what people around me were doing. I learned that I was unable to be in a group without comparing myself, on every level, with people around me. Usually, this resulted in me lowering my opinion of myself. The feelings my first months of Yoga brought up were not by any means all peace and light. I saw, for the first time, how much I was governed my feelings of jealousy, sadness, rage, resentment, and fear. It was a winter of discontent.

But *svadhyaya* is a process that in some ways feels magical. Watching the feelings, I began to have space from them. Over time, I started to have some larger revelations; of how these emotions formed part of a pattern of how I saw myself in relation to the world. And the true miracle of Yogic self-study is that we observe all of our feelings, thoughts, and emotions, whether negative or positive, *without judgment.* It is this that gives us the space to grow. I learned to see my self-judgments, which were constant and negative, as nothing more than thoughts whose power over me was not inevitable. I learned to take a breath before reacting to other people. So many of my words and actions were coming from a dark place; taking a moment before reacting gave me a chance to avoid speaking words that were motivated by anger or jealousy.

Over the years *svadhyaya* has become a more constant practice; from observing mostly myself, on the mat, I have found it becoming a near-constant practice. The process is ongoing. Every day I find moments where I am tightening up, acting because of emotions that are swirling under the surface. I still have plenty of places where I need to soften. But with every year it becomes easier to take the time to speak, and act, from the heart.

Knowledge of our true nature is the wellspring of happiness.

"Is it your wish, my brother, to go into solitude? Is it your wish to seek the way to yourself…Lonely one, you are going the way to yourself. And your way leads past yourself and your seven devils…" Friedrich Nietzsche, in <u>Thus Spake Zarathustra</u>

Listening to the Body

Lately I've been reading a lot of literature on holistic approaches to women's health. One of the best books on the subject is <u>Women's Bodies, Women's Wisdom,</u> by Dr. Christiane Northrup. What struck me most was the idea that many of our illnesses are our souls' way of talking to us. Dr. Northrup sees illness and disease as a sort of last-ditch effort for our souls to let us know what's going on. Usually, the illness is caused by unprocessed memories and emotions from our past that we have 'stuffed down' inside of our bodies in order to not feel their pain. As women, we are subject to this in different ways than men are. We are taught from a young age that only certain types of emotion are acceptable. Depending on the way we were raised, we may believe that our husband and children's happiness comes first. We may never speak some of the 'unacceptable' emotions we feel. I know that when my son was born I felt a lot of things I wasn't supposed to feel. Everyone expected me to be joyous with motherhood. I loved him from the moment of his birth but there was a part of me that mourned my old life, my old body, and my freedom. Luckily I had friends I could share these feelings with, so I didn't just have to swallow them.

Like many holistic practitioners, I believe that emotion and memory are stored in the body. Everything we have ever experienced exists in us somewhere. That's great for those joyous memories, but what happens to the bad stuff? Different emotions cause illness in different parts of the body; for example, repressed creativity can manifest itself as fibroids in the uterus. The body speaks in metaphor. We feel tension in our shoulders and neck from all the emotional weight we carry around. Our lower backs ache from supporting all that we ask it to do.

The material I was reading yesterday excited me. But it didn't penetrate right away. I was exhausted but I wouldn't stop running. In the past 24 hours I had taught 3 yoga classes, run 3 or 4 errands, cleaned house, shoveled snow for an hour, and spent any free moments paying attention to my son. My arm was numb from neck and shoulder tension, and I had pulled muscles in both my legs. Yet after Julian was asleep my heart still raced. There was so much more to do! Laundry to put away, phone calls to return and a chapter to finish writing.

I felt so resistant. My mind kept picturing myself tucked up in bed with a book and American Idol on the television, leaving anything else undone. I was raised to believe that resting was lazy, and that your worth is measured by how hard you work. If I tell my family I am teaching 9 classes a week, they want to know why it's not more. No wonder I have trouble listening to my body; no wonder we all do. Instead of resting when we're tired, we have another cup of coffee or some sugar so we can get our work done. We've lost the art of listening, of going into our bodies and observing what it is we need.

I'm proud to say that last night the message finally penetrated. Instead of finishing my work, I crawled into bed. I turned off the phone. I even put my feet up on a pillow.

Wrestling with time

When I first started practicing yoga, I was in a really big hurry. I wanted to skip past the beginning and go right into the more advanced poses. I started practicing at a gym where many of the students had been practicing for years. It drove me crazy to be unable to do yoga the 'right way'. Part of it was ego; I always want to be good at what I do. But another part was impatience. I remember asking my teacher, week after week, why my hamstrings were still so tight. I couldn't even sit on the floor with my legs stretched out straight. She would always reply that it could take years for my hamstrings to loosen up. Eventually she must have lost patience with me. The last time I asked her she replied, "Why do you care? It doesn't matter." It's one of the wisest things anyone has ever said to me.

I often share this anecdote in yoga classes, especially with beginners. One of the reasons I bring it up is that I need the reminder for myself. It's one of those yoga lessons that has a lot of importance off the mat.

It's so easy to get impatient. We're always in a hurry, we lose our patience, and this wrestling with time carries over into the bigger areas of our lives. Wanting to rush through the grocery line is the same pattern of thought that leads us to rush through everything else. When I was engaged I was impatient to get married. When I was pregnant I couldn't wait for the baby to be born. When I lived in Rome I couldn't wait to be back home. When I was back I was in a hurry to get my yoga certification so I could be a yoga teacher…and it goes on and on. Every time I reached a milestone I barely paused before reaching for the next one.

This constant rushing into the future is a great cause of unhappiness. I can be in a fine mood for days, until I start thinking about all the things I want in the future. I can't wait to have my own home, another baby, a successful teaching career. I can't wait until my college loans are paid off, my husband gets a promotion (or a recording contract), until everything is great and I'm perfectly happy all of the time. As soon as those thoughts begin, I'm snapped out of the moment and into the future. The pleasure of the day is gone and replaced with a sense of what I do not have rather than what I do.

I'm trying to have faith that everything has its own time. Being impatient for things to change won't help anything to change. We are not in complete control over everything that happens to us. When I notice myself spiraling into the future I try to call myself back to the present. I remember that I have enough to eat and a roof over my head, which is fortune enough.

My yoga practice has helped me work towards this faith. I've been trusting that my body will open when it's ready to. Yesterday in a class I watched a student perform a beautiful sequence of asanas; she went from wheel to handstand and back again. Instead of thinking "Wow, I've got to work harder so I can do that", I simply enjoyed the beauty of the postures. Maybe in ten years I'll do that, maybe in twenty, or maybe never. That thought itself was peaceful.

By not pushing my body into the future, I have learned to trust myself. By accepting my body as it is each day, tight or not, I have learned to appreciate it the way it is.

Our bodies, minds, and spirits are opening on their own time, and there's no reason to rush them.

It's All For the Good

Last week in a yoga class I took, the teacher read a story from Swami Satchidananda. I was already meditating on this essay at the time; it was one of those great moments of synchronicity when life gives you what you need. I'll paraphrase the story. There was a king who had a monk to attend him. One day, the monk accidentally cut the king. The monk said, "It's all for the good." The king raged and sent the monk to prison. To which the monk said, "It's all for the good." The king then went hunting one day, and was stalked by a lion. The lion sniffed the king and then wouldn't deign to eat him. The king was thrilled, and went to ask the monk why the lion hadn't killed him. The monk said, "He is the king of beasts as you are a king of men. He wouldn't eat your flesh because of your wound; you were not perfect. I wasn't there because I was in prison; normally I am with you always. If I had been there, he would have eaten me, as I am not wounded. So the cut was for the good, my imprisonment was for the good, it's all for the good."

What would our lives be like if we could take a step back and say, it's all for the good? It's hard to take that distance when you're in the middle of a difficult or painful situation. Sometimes the greater plan is only evident with hindsight.

In 1999 I graduated college. I spent the summer working in a restaurant in a small town in upstate New York. I wasn't ready to let go of my college life. I felt lost. My ambition overwhelmed me; I had no idea if I could make any kind of success of my life. I drank too much, a long relationship was ending, and I was deeply depressed. One night, overtired on a dark country road, I crashed. The car flipped over four or five times. I remember nothing of what happened for about ten minutes before the crash. Somehow I climbed out of the mangled front windshield of the car to start looking for my dog. The paramedics on the scene were expecting me to be dead.

This horrible experience changed everything. For years I had been depressed. Coming close to death snapped me into life. After I could move around again, I went to Italy to visit Mike, to try to work things out. We ended up with Julian. And the injuries I sustained in that car accident are what led me, eventually, to Yoga

When I reflect on that sequence of events, I am filled with wonder. If I hadn't crashed my car, where would I be now? Would something else have snapped me out of my downward spiral, or would I have sunk all the way down? I think the accident was a gift; I believe life works in metaphors. My life was spinning out of control; my car spun out of control.

It's easy to see this with hindsight, a bit harder when you're living through something. If you apply these words, "It's all for the good", to your daily life, like a mantra, you can feel the effect in the present. Sometimes just by meditating on the words you can see the positive benefits a 'negative' situation is having on your own life right now.

I tend to get angry that Mike and I don't own a house. Usually about once a month, I will sulk for a few days that everyone else owns a home while we live with my grandmother, saving money. I wish things would happen more quickly. I try to remember that it's all for the good. Eventually my head clears. My heart lightens. If we owned a home, Mike would probably have to work two jobs. He would not be working on his music and spending time with our son. To help pay bills, I would have to work more and spend less time doing the things I love, spending time with Julian and practicing Yoga. I feel filled with gratitude at how good our lives really are. We may be not be rich but we're sheltered, fed, and clothed. We have loving friends and family, and work that we enjoy. In truth we have everything.

We don't always know why things are for the good, and it's not our job to know. We are not in control of the universe. We don't always know why we've been placed in the lives we're in. When confusion or worry enters your heart, try using these words as your own mantra.

It's all for the good.

The Fruits of Our Labors

"He thought that trying to be the best at wrestling was not what he wanted; also, he knew, it was not likely he could be the best....
And where did he get this idea of wanting to be the best?"

John Irving, <u>The World According to Garp</u>

"Perfectionism—an addiction that afflicts many of us and a web of lies that pervades our culture-is a kind of mask with attractive payoffs...Through a lens tainted with perfectionism, we view things as black and white, either/or, all or nothing...The real perfection is becoming a human being in the same way a tree is a tree."

Vimala McClure, <u>A Woman's Guide to Tantra Yoga</u>

"Everybody who has ever felt a moment of arrogance knows that arrogance is just a cover-up for really feeling that you're the worst horse, and always trying to prove other-wise."

Pema Chodron, <u>The Wisdom of No Escape</u>

Teaching Yoga scares me. Every time I'm beginning a class, I feel the adrenaline course through my veins. Panicky thoughts fly through my head. So many things can go wrong; my biggest fear is that during a class I will just stop. I fear my nerves will get the best of me and I will freeze, unable to speak another word. I take a deep breath and go on. As my nerves seem to keep getting worse, I have been engaged in *svadhyaya* (self-study), to try to root out the problem.

And what it comes down to, I think, is perfectionism. Every time I teach a class I want it to be a perfect class, the best class ever. As always in Yoga, an issue that's been part of my life for as long as I can remember has shown up on the mat. It's less of an issue in my own practice; after four years I've made peace with doing the pose that is available to me in the moment. But with teaching it's harder. My actions affect how others will think of me, and that's scary.

In the past perfectionism served a purpose in my life. In college it drove me to earn perfect grades, to write the best papers, to make the best comments in discussions. In my working life it made me efficient. I never missed days of work. I always was promoted. Yet all of those little victories were so empty. When I received an A paper back I always felt hollow. The grade was an anticlimax; nothing was ever enough. Compliments from bosses and co-workers were the same. There was a moment's pleasure followed by some nameless feeling of okay, so now what?

This is the lure of perfectionism. It distorts all of our efforts; we are not doing the work for its own sake, but doing it for the sake of perfection, of doing the best job. We may procrastinate. Sometimes it's hard to get started when you know your best efforts will never be good enough. Perfectionism breeds anxiety and bleeds out true enjoyment. The quest to do something perfectly takes us out of ourselves and out of the moment. We are attached to the fruits of our labor rather than the labors themselves. Action undertaken in the hope of an external reward very rarely satisfies. If we are doing something in the hope of approval from others, we will always fail. After the compliments have faded from our ears, we are still left with ourselves. If we don't have our own approval, we will be back where we started, ready to take up the next task in the quest for reward.

How do we escape the lure of the perfect? I find peace in the idea of Karma Yoga. One of the meanings of Karma Yoga is to dedicate the fruits of one's labors to God, to go through the work with no attachment to the outcome, but with the utmost attention to the work itself. In this way we still give the best of ourselves, but we keep our attention focused on the task, not the results of the task. We can apply this idea to every action we take. Not everyone believes in a higher power; you can still ease your way out of perfectionism by coming back to the work itself, focusing your mind on what you are doing. The mat is a place to begin work on this. We learn to stop comparing ourselves to others. We learn that in asana practice, there is no perfection other than what is.

I find it helpful to try to keep my ego out of it. I remember that when I am teaching Yoga, it has very little to do with me. I am passing down knowledge that comes from others, and the students are learning because of their own openness to the knowledge. I think this applies to all things we work at; our ego is a hindrance rather than a help. Perfectionism is part of the lie of our separateness. The perfectionist part of us cries, "Me! I did that!" When really it's not so. All of our skills, all of the talents we have, are a result of the lives we have lived and the people who have intermingled with us along the way. Every person we have met on our path has helped to create us, as we have helped to create them.

Learning to Read

Julian is learning to read. Watching this process is amazing. Since he was in the womb, we've been reading to him. While I was pregnant, I read to him from whatever book I happened to be reading. As soon as he could focus his eyes, we started with baby books. Every day of his life, we took time out to read to him. We've waited eagerly for the time when he would be able to read for himself.

Now, before our eyes, a process has begun that seems to spring from deep inside of him. Over the past few months, he's become more and more interested in words. Lately, the pace has accelerated. He constantly asks us to spell things for him. He reads the words he knows while we are enjoying his nighttime story. He picks up pens and pencils and writes in his beautiful, straggly handwriting.

To me, the most amazing thing about the process is how little we have to do with it. It reminds me of how he learned to speak; he started with babbles, and suddenly he was learning ten new words a day. His curiosity was unquenchable. It's as if there is a force within him compelling him toward growth. It's unstoppable. We aren't prodding him into any of these activities; he is the one who is so eager to learn.

I have felt this within myself lately. For the past year I've been a little obsessive over a few aspects of my practice. I've spent a lot of time worrying about being unable to meditate. Every time I tried, I grew anxious. My breath got shorter, my heart started to pound, and things spiraled until I gave up. During class meditations I would just try to relax, unable to even follow the words of the teacher. Eventually I gave up; I decided that asana was enough meditation for me, and maybe in a few years I'd be able to sit for meditation practice.

A few weeks ago I started to feel a new urge. I began craving a few minutes of silence, sitting in lotus. I tried it and for the first time felt okay in mediation, okay with sitting with a quiet mind. Every few days now I feel the desire to meditate; I've tried a few different ways, figuring out the practices that feel best for me. I can only sit for a few minutes, but the desire is there along with the ability. And it didn't come until I began to trust that when I was ready, I would be able to sit.

We all have this force inside of us, this yearning to grow. The most important thing we can do is just let go and allow ourselves to unfold. This to me, is what grace means. We prepare the soil of ourselves. We plant the seeds. And the force of life takes care of the rest. All we have to do is trust it.

The Tyranny of Expectations

In yoga, we are trying to come back to the present moment. We are trying to see through the illusions created by our conscious, monkey-like minds, in order to live in truth and see with clarity. We start out simply observing our minds. Soon we notice that we are not often in the present; our minds flit back and forth between future and past, and when we are in the present our attention is often not in the physical space we inhabit. Our minds have wandered out of the room. It is this constant thinking into the future that creates expectations. We have certain preconceived ideas about what is going to happen in the next hour, day, and month. Our minds are constantly jumping ahead, and this limits how we live in the present.

Over the past few years, I've found it much easier to stay in the present moment. At first it only happened during Yoga class, but over time it came off the mat as well. I thought I was doing pretty well about living in the present, and staying open to the future.

I truly believe that life always puts in our path exactly what we need to learn. A few weeks ago, my husband and I got some scary news from my doctor. A screening test on the baby came up positive; there was a chance our baby had a lethal birth defect.

Well. Aside from the shock, and the worry, I came up against the tyranny of expectation. After an easy and uncomplicated pregnancy with my first son, the last thing I expected was any kind of complication with this one. The whole time I have thought of myself as open to life, to whatever happens, I was much more rigid than I realized. In my head I had a very firm idea about what my pregnancy would mean. I would work my normal schedule, keep up my normal yoga practice, and do everything I do while not pregnant, all while carrying a perfectly healthy baby. Every time my mind had jumped ahead to the future, this is what it had laid out for itself. Even though on some level I feared, like all expectant parents, some kind of complication, I did have a preconceived idea of what the future would hold.

We waited five long days for the test results that told us our new baby didn't have this lethal birth defect. I felt stripped down and naked. Because of the amniocentesis, I was ordered to take a break from exercising and physical activity. So I couldn't work, and when it snowed I couldn't even shovel. I wasn't allowed to do yoga asana, which is where I feel most grounded and connected. My husband yelled at me every time I got out of bed. My routine, which is very particular, was completely destroyed. Many of the things that make up what I think of as myself were taken away.

I observed my mind trying to create new expectations, new patterns of thoughts. If the baby has it, this will happen, and this and this…For five days I tried, as hard as I could, to keep my mind empty. I tried not to push scary thoughts away; I cried when I needed to, and talked with my husband and family and friends. But I worked, whenever I was silent, on breathing. Every time thoughts of the future came into my head I simply reminded myself that we *didn't know,* and there was no way to know, and there was nothing to do but wait. It was, in a way, easier to let go because we had no control over the situation. The only thing I could control was my attitude toward the baby, no matter what the end result would be. So when I started to get anxious, I would bring my attention back to my breath, to breathing deeply into my belly, deeply enough to rock and soothe the baby in my womb. For those moments, I was free of expectations about the test results

When we got the good news that baby didn't have this birth defect, it took a while for life to snap back into place. My expectations that the baby was okay had turned out to be right; yet something had shifted in my mind, or spirit. It was too late to go back to the same routine, to feeling the same way about my life and my pregnancy. We can't know what will happen. So far the baby is okay, and the abnormal test result was probably caused my severe case of hypoglycemia. But even with all back to normal, I don't think I'll go back to feeling the way I did before. I'm going to keep on working on staying in the present, free of any expectations about what the next few months (or indeed, the rest of my life) will bring.

Enough is Enough

We have entered the season of gifts. For the next month, we will be ceaselessly bombarded with messages exhorting us to buy. Conversations will revolve around our holiday shopping—is it done yet? How much have you spent? What are you hoping to get? Television, newspapers, radios, the Internet, billboards...all will be filled with advertisements imploring us to spend and buy, spend and buy.

There is nothing wrong with giving gifts. For the giver, there is pleasure in choosing a present that will make someone's face light up. And when you receive a gift someone has chosen for you with thought and intent, you feel the love and intention of the giver

One of the *yamas* (ethical precepts) of Yoga is *aparigraha,* which is usually translated as greedlessness. Vimala McLure writes, "To choose *Aparigraha* is to choose an outer life that is as much in harmony with our inner values as possible. To choose simplicity is to reduce the quantity while increasing the quality. It is to face the disease of greed as it has insidiously permeated our lives, and to make a daily commitment to its healing." Can we integrate *aparigraha* into our holidays? The message of our culture is the opposite of *aparigraha.* We are constantly being told that we don't have enough. The message is always to want more and better; a fancier cell phone, a bigger television, better clothing and accessories. One practice is to truly think about the gifts you are buying. Are you purchasing something just so you can cross that name off your list? Are you making choices in your buying that are good for the environment, and good for your spirit? One thing to consider is consumable gifts—lovely foodstuffs, gift certificates for massages or yoga classes.

In many religions, the winter holidays were originally a celebration of light at the darkest time of year. This is also a time for reflection and evaluation, a time for counting our blessings and preparing for the next growing season. Use this time to take stock of your physical environment. What is in your home that is too much, that is more than enough? There are many charities that are eager for goods that to you just may be clutter. Keeping aparigraha in mind, we can find a balance between giving and receiving. We already have so much.

"We are always afraid that there will not be enough…Instead of seeing our riches and giving generously to other, we become nothing more than rich beggars, always asking for more…." B.K.S. Iyengar, <u>*Light on Life*</u>

Season of Wonder

Every morning that weather permits, the baby and I walk my older son, Julian, to school. It's a short walk, only about ten minutes, through pleasant suburban streets. There's something wonderful about taking the same walk every day. It's much easier to observe changes in the life around us as we pass the same spots, day after day. Back in March, Julian and I started searching for signs of spring. We challenged each other to find five signs of spring on those cold days when there was still snow on the ground, and the skies were gray. We noticed melting snow, returning birds, a hint of warmth in the air, baby buds on the trees, and the first leaves of crocuses just popping up, surrounded by snow that was still unmelted.

Day by day we've charted the progress of the advancing season. Three weeks ago there were just buds on the trees. Tuesday morning we walked to school, and on some of the trees, there they were. Baby leaves, tiny and perfect. We've watched the blossoms on the plum and dogwood trees fall off and be replaced by leaves. Dandelions are everywhere.

A few days ago Julian swatted at a fat bumblebee that flew near us. I told him, casually, (which is sometimes the best way for a parent to convey important information), that bees were important. He was silent and I could almost feel his thinking, trying to process the idea that these flying, stinging bugs, which really scare him, could be important. Finally he asked why. So I told him about pollination; how bees travel the neighborhood, helping the flowers to continue to flower. I told him that thanks to the bees, in a few years the pear trees that line our street may bear fruit. In the quiet of my mind I felt my own heart lift at how perfectly the bee fits into the work of nature.

Even the baby is in awe of Spring. Every time we go out he looks in wonder at the leaves, yelling, "Look! Look!" Of course, it sounds more like "Dook!" but that in itself in something to listen to in wonder. I hadn't realized he was aware enough to notice how different the world is looking these days. For most of the time he has been conscious of the outside world, the trees have been bare. Observing a baby open to the world and become connected is an awesome thing.

We serve ourselves well when we cultivate wonder. We open our hearts every time we pause and take in the glory that is. What better way is there to inoculate ourselves against boredom and despair? Let yourself be in awe of the beauty you find in yourself, in other people, in things natural and in things made by human hands.

"During my years as a psychotherapist felt that people…were suffering from a deeper malaise. They had fallen out of love with life itself, which, in their adult years, had become an absorbing collection of problems.

The soul has different concerns, of equal value: downtime for reflection, conversation, and reverie; beauty that is captivating and pleasuring; relatedness to the environs and to people; and an animal's rhythm of rest and activity." Thomas Moore, in <u>The Reenchantment of Everyday Life</u>

Meeting Resistance

Imagine yourself flowing through an asana practice, enjoying the movements and the breath. Suddenly you feel as if you've hit a wall. Your breath loses its rhythm, your muscles tighten. Your mind stiffens and snaps out of 'Yoga' and back into your everyday stream of consciousness. You've hit a block, either emotional or physical. We meet resistance when we leave our comfort zone and push out into the great beyond.

Or maybe you never make it to the mat at all. You've been practicing for a while, and suddenly you just can't do it. You find all sorts of excuses for skipping your practice. You're tired; you have too many errands to run. Your mind is capable of coming up with all sorts of reasons not to practice.

If you have been to a few yoga classes, you may have heard your teacher refer to 'resistance'. As you practice, paying attention to your emotions, there will be times when you feel as if you can't practice anymore. Resistance expresses itself in different ways. Writers call it writer's block. Resistance crops up in every field of endeavor.

In Yoga asana it may run up as resentment towards a particular pose, certain teachers, or just wanting some time off to focus on something else.

Resistance crops up when we leave our comfort zone and try to grow. Organisms look for homeostasis. The familiar, the stable, is much easier and more natural than trying to change. In yoga asana, the poses we are most emotionally resistant to are the ones we need the most. It serves us well to persist in them. They have the most to teach us.

When I began my yoga practice I was hampered by tight hamstrings and lower back. Sitting in *dandasana* and bending forward in paschimottanasana (sitting forward fold) were moments of agony and torture. My legs were bent almost in half when I tried to sit on the floor. Whenever the teacher called for these poses I groaned. Luckily, pride wouldn't let me just sit them out. I took great care to do them, safely. I tried to take in the teacher's words that 'it didn't matter how straight my legs were." My encounter with *paschimottanasana* taught me more in the first year of practice than any of the poses I did well. I took to heart my teacher's advice to watch your reaction to each pose. I noticed that most of reaction had to do with pride rather than pain. I could deal with pain; I had been through 11 hours of natural childbirth. And I truly wanted to open my body, thus I was willing to sit with the discomfort. As I went through these poses, week after week, I noticed that what hurt was being 'no good'. So much of my personality was invested in being 'good' at things. I tended to quit things I wasn't good at to avoid criticism. I stuck with anything where I could achieve. I had enough strength and flexibility to do well in the standing postures, which is why it hurt so much to be unable to do these poses. Every time I sat with my bent knees in *dandasana*, I felt like a failure. Through patience and persistence my legs began to open up. Also through patience, I began to observe my ego's reactions during class. With time, I was able to feel compassion for myself, and detach a little from the judging. My imperfect *dandasana* taught me more than my 'perfect' triangles.

Resistance doesn't go away. You deal with it in one place and it will crop up somewhere else. I no longer cringe when asked to sit on the floor with straight legs. Lately my resistance is coming up in regard to headstand. I have this idea that since I am a yoga teacher, I have no right to teach yoga unless I can do headstand in the middle of the room. In group classes I groan when it's headstand time. I am embarrassed at my headstand. It's my *dandasana* issue all over again, but this time I know how to deal with it.

The first thing to do when you encounter resistance to to notice it. When you are feeling resistant to going to class, check in with yourself. Acknowledge your resistance to the practice. Is it really resistance, or are you just tired? Are you menstruating, or stressed-out? If your body is too tired, maybe it's just fatigue. But if not, maybe you have found your edge. Maybe something happened in your last class that didn't seem to affect you at the time, but you've been stewing through unconsciously.

The process of hatha yoga brings up emotions and memories stored in the body. The mat is a mirror and through self-study we come to know our selves. We don't always like what we see. Yes, yoga is relaxing, but the process of opening your body and spirit is sometimes a painful one. On the mat we meet ourselves.

Resistance to the practice and the poses often comes just when we are about to make a major leap in our understanding, The next time you encounter resistance, meet it head on. Acknowledge it, examine it, and proceed anyway.

Ebb and Flow

I will begin by saying that I love summer. I love the heat, the sun, the green of the trees. I love the freedom to run out of the house unencumbered by coat and hat and even shoes. I love the beach, I love the lush, verdant life of a forest in August. I love to practice Yoga in the heat of the day, when the heat melts tightness away, and the sweat takes all that is not needed out of my body.

I can't say I'm happy about the change of the seasons. I can appreciate the coming of autumn; I can look forward to the holidays. But already I feel my summer Yoga practice (which I'm awfully attached to!) transforming. My muscles are tighter. It's taking longer to build heat. No more hundred-degree heat doing half the work for me! I'm starting to feel anxious about the long winter to come. How will I keep two little kids happy without trips to the park? How will I get two little kids dressed in coats, mittens, hats, and boots to even step outside? Will the dark invite depression? Already I'm living in the future, waiting for the spring that is seven months away. It's certainly not very Yogic.

Patanjali warns us, in the Yoga Sutras (Chapter 2, Sutra 3) of the obstacles to enlightenment. "These obstacles—the causes of man's sufferings—are ignorance, egoism, attachment, aversion, and the desire to cling to life." I'm certainly attached to summer, with an aversion to winter, and I would cling forever to the summer, if I could. Bearing the teachings of Yoga in mind, I'm trying to flow with the changes the season brings. In my asana practice, which was physically very vigorous throughout the summer, I'm becoming more focused on what's happening mentally. I'm striving to appreciate this cooler weather, and enjoy the different rhythms of the school year.

Making peace with what we don't like doesn't mean repressing our emotions. What it does mean is taking that lovely step back into the witness mind. I will try to step back into the quiet center that lies behind the torrents of thoughts, emotions, and sensory stimuli that fluctuate in my consciousness. The more time we spend in the quiet mind, in this place of Yoga, the more we can enjoy the ebb and the flow of life. Everything changes; nothing is still. Our moods, our physical states, our relationships, all are in a constant state of flux. The more we trust in the cycles of life and the constant oscillation of the universe, the more we can be open to the joy that is present in every moment.

Learning to Fall

When Julian, my older son, learned to walk, he took off like a racehorse from a starting gate. From the moment he could take a few steps alone, he just ran. He couldn't balance, so he had to keep moving as fast as he could. Needless to say, he fell a lot, and his first year of walking involved lots of bumps to the head. It was exhilarating to watch his sheer determination to enjoy the wonders of motion.

My second son, Kai, is a different story. For two months now, when people have asked if he could walk, I haven't been sure how to answer. Could he walk? Sure. But most of the time he chose not to. He's been taking steps for over a month, but he doesn't like to fall. He's a super fast crawler, so I guess the risk involved in walking didn't seem worth it. His first few weeks of walking were very amusing. He held his hands out in front of him, rather like Frankenstein's monster. If he started to fall, he did a preemptive drop onto his bottom, nicely cushioned by his diaper. Unlike most new walkers, he's only bumped his head twice while learning to walk. There are benefits to caution.

Thinking about these two approaches to walking has of course made me think of Yoga asana practice, in particular, inversions. We yogis run the gamut from caution to fearlessness when it comes to trying the new and challenging. I've seen brand new beginners, ignoring cautions from teachers, throw themselves into headstand or handstand the first time they see the pose, without a thought for their own safety. Sometimes they fall pretty hard; other times the effort is rewarded with success. I think of Julian, who a month or two after learning to walk, took off at a run at our county park. He made it all the way into the duck pond before I caught him.

Some of us yogis take our time, working patiently on the prep poses for months or even years. Sometimes we are truly not ready for a pose, and what's holding us back is justifiable caution. Other times our bodies are ready, our minds are not. I think of Kai, taking one more step every day, hands in front of him to brace his fall.

Can we find the balance between cautiousness and fearlessness? We need both elements in our asana practice (and our lives as well!) Caution keeps us safe. We take the time to know our bodies and prepare them for more advanced asana.

And then, we need a little bit of fearlessness—or call it courage—to make the leap.

The Only Way Out is Through

The words above are a mantra that popped into my head a few months ago. I don't know if I read the phrase somewhere, or it just arrived out of the ether. Either way, it became a lodestone; something to hold onto during moments of stress. When you first meditate on those words, comfort is the last thing you would expect from them. The only way out is through; meaning, there is no escape, in that moment, from your particular situation. Scary words, but wise ones.

When I was deep in labor with Kai, those words came back to me. As anyone who's been through childbirth can tell you, it's pretty painful. The first time I gave birth, the pain terrified me. Rather than going with the pain, I fought it. I tried as hard as I could *not* to feel what I was feeling. The whole experience was frightening and stressful. Yet at the end, when it was obvious the baby was coming and the pain wasn't going to kill me, I actually enjoyed the experience. In the five years after my first birth, I often longed to do it again. I didn't just want to have another baby, but to go through the experience of labor and birth in a different way.

As I prepared to have my new baby, nothing prepared me better for the birth than what I have learned through Yoga practice. This time, when the pain got intense, I remembered to breathe. Rather than fighting the pain of each contraction, I felt it, keeping the thought in my head that the pain was working to get my baby out. And always, that phrase, the only way out is through.

After baby, I used the mantra even more. One day I was at the end of my rope. Kai was only a few days old. He was nursing constantly and my nipples were cracked and bleeding. The pain of feeding him was so intense that I would prefer to be in labor. I was experiencing post-birth contractions that were easily as painful as labor itself, every single time he fed. I had barely slept more than an hour at a stretch in a good two months, due to the discomforts of pregnancy. I took a nice hot shower, finally feeling some of the pain ebb, relaxed because he was sleeping. As I dried off I heard his wail of hunger from the bedroom. My own tears came. I just couldn't stand the thought of going back to him, loving his little self yet being in so much pain as he ate. Once again the phrase came into my head, and I felt it's true weight. There was no choice but for me to suffer. I couldn't ignore the screaming baby; newborns need to eat whenever they want to. I couldn't stop nursing him and give him artificial baby milk because it's not an option for our family. I couldn't just stay in the bathroom and hide. The only thing to do was to face the pain. The only way out is through.

So I unlocked the bathroom door, and went to nurse my baby. The pain was excruciating, but I remembered to breathe. That moment felt like a watershed for me. I don't think I have ever been as miserable as I was in that moment, knowing that I had no choice but to go back to Kai, despite my own pain.

The thing is, I don't think I could have done it without Yoga. At least not in the same way. What many people who have never practiced don't realize is that Yoga is uncomfortable. Sometimes it hurts! Not in a bad, injury-causing kind of way, but in a muscles being stretched that haven't stretched since you were five kind of way. It doesn't just hurt in the beginning; it continues to hurt, because we are constantly playing to the edge of our own abilities. But that's the only way to grow.

The difference is how we are learning to react or rather, not react. When your teacher comes and deepens your stance a little in warrior II, so now your front bottom thigh is protesting at being asked to work harder, and your arms are getting tired because you've been holding the pose for what feels like ten minutes, and maybe even your neck is getting tired of holding your head up, but you *stay in the pose anyway,* because you're not doing something dangerous, it's just your body rebelling at being asked to work harder, you learn you are committed to the practice. And the only way out is through.

And that's what makes the difference. We work hard; we challenge ourselves, because we are committed to our own growth and our own self-discovery. There's no easy way out. I see the Yoga journey as being a quest, a quest for truth and bliss and contentment and joy. And the sad part is that sometimes it's easier to give up, to just stay home and watch TV, to let the practice slip, because the truth is that you have to wade through a lot of dark stuff on your way to Yoga; all the lies you've ever told to yourself, all the horrible ways you've behaved in your life, all the bad stuff you've done as well as the good. The mat is like a mirror, and sometimes the reflection that you see isn't very pretty. But we stick with it, because the destination is worth it. We are happier, kinder, calmer—maybe even a little wiser. And there's no other way to get there than by doing the work. The only way out is through.

Forward bends and the art of surrender.

In Yoga we view the state of the body as a metaphor for the state of the mind, the heart, and the spirit. Rather, all of these divisions serve as metaphors for each other. Even more accurately, the state of the body is the state of the mind is the state of the heart is the state of the spirit. There is no division. We are one with ourselves.

Slumped shoulders? Depression. Shoulders pulled up to the ears? An almost unbearable inner tension. Shallow breathing? Stress. An observant observer can pick up many clues to the people one watches just by looking at the shape of their body.

When we practice our asana, we are changing the shape of our body and thus the condition of our mind.

So forward bends. They are a sticky point for many an aspiring yogi. They are very difficult for beginners. Years of walking, sitting, aerobics, and sports have often tightened the hamstrings to the point where there is almost no flexibility in the lower back. Most adults, even those who are very active, cannot bring their hands anywhere near the floor when asked to bend over to touch their toes.

As the hamstrings (the muscles at the backs of the legs) tighten, all sorts of other things happen to the body. Tight hamstrings tend to pull the sacrum and the bottom of the spine down toward the floor, skewing the alignment of the lower back. This throws everything else in the spine out of alignment, leading to discomfort, which leads to more tightening up, which leads to more tension. Unless, of course, something breaks the cycle.

I remember my first year of practice and the memory stings. I felt shame that first year. I hated myself for my tightness. My body was no more than something I raged at. What hurts most now is the memory of how attached I was to the idea of being the best, as if my self was so weak that the only way I could feel worthy of existence was if I outshone everyone else. Now I feel grateful for my first teacher; her kindness, her attention. She gave me attention even though I wasn't the best, and that sparked the idea that maybe she thought I was worth paying attention to.

In forward bends it is easy to compare your pose to everyone else's. If the class is sitting on the floor in *paschimottanasana*, it is easy to see where you fit into the class. Maybe your hamstrings are as tight as violin strings. Maybe years of running and walking and sitting and cringing have tightened the back of your body so much that you can't sit with your legs straight out without extreme discomfort. Those hamstrings have been contracting upon themselves for years; they don't even remember how to release. There's no way to hide where you are.

I would look at myself in my forward bends and wince. For years I was an avid exerciser. Even during my pregnancy I walked for almost an hour a day. My legs were strong and very tight. I had never bothered to take the time to stretch. I came to yoga as a very sad, very angry, 23 year old woman. My body was tight as a drum. I was holding on to so much scary stuff. I had abused my body for years with drugs, alcohol, cigarettes, and over-exercising, and there was no way my body trusted me enough to let go.

In forward bending there is more than one type of surrender.

The first one is that of your ego. For the bend to feel good, and safe, you have to let go of any ideas you have about how far you are going to stretch. The first time my instructor asked us to sit on the floor, stretch our legs out, and bend forward, I was in for a shock. My mind had me with my face on my knees, blissful like the other yoginis in the room. Reality had me with legs that wouldn't straighten at all, and a stabbing pain in my lower back when I tried to move even a millimeter forward.

If you're an overachiever, if you're a perfectionist, if your self-worth is tied only to what you can accomplish, learning to surrender your ideas of yourself is a very important part of your practice.

During those first months of practice I would continually ask Carrie, "When will my hamstrings open up?" Her answers varied. "It can take years." And finally, the most important answer. "Does it matter?"

It did matter to me. Being young and strong I progressed quickly through many of the asanas. As a former martial artist, the warrior poses were familiar and comfortable. I had the drive to improve. I was carrying 50 pounds of baby weight, and very depressed. Yoga was the only light in the tunnel, the only way I could see out of the darkness, so I threw myself into the practice. My hamstrings would not loosen.

Not only did I want to save my own life, I wanted to be "good at yoga". I still thought these was a prize to be won for being the best in the class, as if there was a yoga grand champion of the world which I could aspire to be one day. My class-mates were all my competitors. (I don't take all the blame for that one; we women are raised to compete against each other). It was as if I thought getting my head to my knees in *paschimottanasana* would give me the love and admiration I constantly needed to keep filling the empty space inside of me.

It took a year for me to give up on my hamstrings. It took a year to notice that I couldn't calm my mind because of the constant shrilling of my ego, which demanded so much of me. "You're heavier than her. She's prettier than you. Why are you so weak?" During that year, despite two or three classes a week, my ham-strings barely opened at all. My heels were still way off the floor in down dog, my knees were still bent whenever I bent forward, but I decided it didn't matter.

And they began to open up.

About six months ago, I noticed that sometimes my heels do touch the floor in down dog. Some days, I can bend forward with straight legs without pain in my lower back.

And you know what? It still doesn't matter.

The second type of surrender I've discovered through forward bending is more subtle. It can only be felt when some of the ego stuff has been dealt with. When the go has stopped its relentless bids for attention, and the mind is able to quiet a little, there is time to listen. There is a chance to hear the Self, and the seductive whisper of surrendering, just a little bit, to your life as it is. It's some-thing I noticed a few months ago, when my asana practice was slowing down. I was working in an office 25 hours a week and taking care of my son and our home the rest of the time. It didn't leave much time for asana. When I got Julian to sleep I was too tired to think of practicing. I was only getting to one class a week, and one teacher training session a month.

Yet I was practicing. I was practicing *uttanasana* (standing forward fold). I was doing this pose about 20 times a day, without even noticing it.

Julian was 3 at the time. I spent a lot of time picking up after him. I began to take a few moments, after reaching down to pick up a toy, to just stay there. I'd take a deep breath or two, my legs would release, and I'd hear a chain of pops coming from my upper back. I'd feel the rush of blood to my head, and rise up feeling a little bit better.

At around the same time I began to notice a change in my mental attitude. I'd been fighting my life for a long, long time, but never so hard as the past few years.

I wasn't really aware of my rage. I raged at the limitations of motherhood. I raged at myself for 'screwing up my life' by having a baby right out of college. I raged at my husband. I raged at the fact that we were in debt, with no home of our own, with no chance of things changing for a good long time.

About two months after my intensive forward bending began, I began to notice a change in my attitude. I started to feel more accepting. Thoughts would come into my head but now they were gentler. Yes, I was stuck living at home, the place I had never wanted to come back to. But my Grandmother isn't well; when she is gone, won't we treasure these years together? Yes, we owe a lot of money for our educations. But those were the best years of my life, and the brain I have now was formed by those years. My husband is what he is. He is not mine to control. He is as God made him.

Every time I bent forward I could hear a voice. "Surrender to the will of God." The meaning is clear even if you don't like the word god. Surrender to the flow of life. Surrender to your nature. Surrender to nature. Surrender to what is. Let go. Stop fighting and go with the current.

This idea of surrender is one I have been thinking of a great deal lately. For many years I experienced chronic depression. If you knew me only as an acquaintance you would be shocked. On the whole I appear cheerful and friendly. Underneath I denounced myself, doubt myself, and hate myself.

For ten years I worked to pull myself out of this depression, which was more of a meta-depression; a darkness that had been present for as long as I could remember. More than a depression, it is an idea of myself formed by circumstances. I see myself as worthless, evil, mean, alone, unlovable, abandoned or about to be abandoned, and unlovable.

I tried to kill these feelings with drugs, alcohol, exercise, sex, relationships, overwork, and academic rigor. Some of these techniques were more successful than others. Some almost killed me, over and over.

When my son was born I had the most powerful reason in the world to try to save myself. When I found Yoga six months after Julian's birth, I found a tool that wouldn't kill me or make me worse. A year after starting practice I told a friend, who had known me through many of the bad times, that I thought I needed this practice. That it would be an anchor that could ground me through the rest of my life. It has done that; there was a glimmer of strength in me that clung to the practice, even as I continued to smoke cigarettes and sabotage my relationship and just generally ruin my life. Over time the strong part of me, the part that wanted to live, was fed by the practice and grew stronger. The most I was hoping for, at the beginning of my practice, was something that would help me live my life without going crazy and living in depression. I never thought that through the practice I would find myself and a way to live in joy.

My main point is this. A few weeks ago I had one of my bad days. My good days outnumber the bad now, but the bad days are still as bad as they ever were. Death wins out over life. I feel like I'm walking through murky water. Horrible fears fill me. The fears turn to anger and I hate everyone. I can barely be a competent parent to my son. I snap at everyone else. Usually it's hard to remember that these moods pass. But on my last bad day I heard a voice in my head. The voice said, "Put your faith in the practice."

I relaxed. My psychic pressure eased. The practice will not conquer death. The practice will not solve my money problems. The practice will not magically make me a happy secure person instantly. But if I practice regularly, I will regain my perspective. In the short term, I will stop panicking. In the long term, I have seen what the practice has done for people. The yogis I know are not saints or angels. But they always seem peaceful, and their warmth envelops you when you speak with them. They seem comfortable in their own skins.

Put your faith in the practice, the voice said, and I relaxed. My heart leapt. For a moment I had a bright shining hope that this Yoga would keep me on a healthy path.

My life is my path and my only job is to surrender to it.

Surrender to the practice. If you've lived your whole life without faith, try having faith in the practice.

The Eight Limbs of Yoga

Meet The Yamas

The Yoga Sutras of Patanjali are generally considered the blueprint for modern yoga philosophy. Scholars believe that Patanjali (whose identity is shrouded by history, and who in fact may been more than one person) created the <u>Sutras</u> to collect and codify the wisdom of Yoga that comes to us from older texts, such as the <u>Vedas</u>, the <u>Upanishads</u>, and the <u>Bhagavad-Gita</u>. In the Sutras we are given the eight limbs of yoga practice, meaning disciplines, or the actions one performs to become a yogi. First, we'll take a look at the first limb, the *Yamas*, or abstentions.

One of the interesting things about the *Yamas* is that they are a list of don'ts; they are the behaviors we should avoid if we hope to progress along our spiritual path. But being things we shouldn't do, the <u>Yamas</u> carry their own opposite within them. By knowing how we shouldn't behave, it becomes equally clear how we should.

The first *yama*, which is the root of all the others, is *ahimsa*, or non-harming. Sometimes it is translated also as nonviolence, but ahimsa refers to more than violence. Georg Feurstein writes, "It consists in unconditional nonmaliciousness toward all beings at all times and in all situations." This includes the self. When we are in doubt on how to behave in a particular situation, we can always come back to the rule of ahimsa.

Our next yama is *satya*, or truthfulness. We should invite *satya* into our lives not just on a superficial level, avoiding obvious lies and deceptions, but also on a deeper level. Perhaps we begin to notice that aspects of the way we live are a distortion of our true selves. We bring *satya* into relationships with others, with ourselves, and with the world at large.

The third yama is *asteya*, or non-stealing. Through self-examination we begin to observe where we seek to take that which does not belong to us. In this context, taking more than we need and wasting resources is stealing.

Next comes *brahmacarya,* to follow god. In earlier times *brahmacarya* was interpreted to mean chastity. In large part this was because sex goes hand in hand with attachment and with following desire, inevitably clouding the mind. Most modern yogis are 'householders', meaning we are in and of the world, and chastity is not something we can reasonably practice (particularly if we are already married!). Modern commentators thus shed a different light on this yama, choosing instead to see it as a call to discipline and restraint in how we live our lives and spend our eneregy.

The final yama is *aparigraha*, or greedlessness, which shares much with *asteya*. How often do we eat when we are already full? How much of our energy goes towards earning more money so we can buy more stuff?

Unlike a great deal of Western philosophy, Yoga philosophy is eminently practical. These disciplines are not lofty ethical precepts, but practices meant to be the guiding forces in our daily lives. We can start by integrating the *Yamas* into our Hatha, or physical, Yoga practice. The mat, as always, can serve as a microcosm of the rest of our lives. Below are some questions to meditate on to help bring the *Yamas* into your practice.

1. *Ahimsa* starts with the self. Do you hurt yourself in your Yoga practice, by pushing too hard or even practicing too much? How much kindness and love do you offer yourself in your Yoga practice? What kind of thoughts do you direct to others in the class?

2. *Asteya*, or non-stealing, is easy to observe on a physical level—just don't take what doesn't belong to you. Can you find a way to apply asteya and aparigraha, greedlessness, to your practice? Do you seek more attention than you need? Do you always try to be in the front of the room, the better to get the teacher's attention? Do you have an attitude of greed toward your practice, always seeking to achieve more, including asanas your body may not be ready for?

3. *Satya*. Do you have an attitude of truthfulness towards yourself in your yoga practice? Do you honor the days when you are tired? Do you give your best and truest effort and discipline to the practice?

4. *Brahmacarya*. What is the goal of your yoga practice? If you are not comfortable with the idea of god, the yama still applies. To what are you dedicating your efforts? Do you seek to improve yourself for the good of the world, and for the good you can do as a balanced, happy person?

After Yama, Niyama

So we come to the second limb of the eightfold path: *niyama*. Often, we call *yama* and *niyama* the 'dos and don'ts' of yoga ethics. But there is a more subtle difference. The *yamas* deal with the relationship of self to the outside world, giving us useful guidelines to follow in our intercourse with society. The *niyamas*, or observances, deal more with the relationship of the self to the self. The practices detailed in *niyama* lead us further along the path to Yoga.

First is *shaoca*, usually translated as cleanliness. Being a Yogic concept, this encompasses more than just the surface level of having a clean skin and even a clean living area. *Shaoca* is also sometimes translated as clarity. It speaks to a universal truth; that the state of our mind is reflected by what is around us. In the physical world we can honor shaoca by cleaning and decluttering our surroundings. Who among us can think clearly when all around us is chaos? We bring *shaoca* then into our physical body; we eat fresh, healthy food, contributing to clean insides. We practice hatha yoga to detoxify our bodies. We practice meditation or concentration to clarify our minds.

Santosa follows *shaoca*. *Santosa* is usually translated from the Sanskrit as 'contentment'. This in itself is a lovely word, but there is more to the meaning. Sanskrit is a language that was designed to communicate spiritual truths; therefore, it often takes more than one English word to translate the concept. A fuller explanation of *santosa* is 'acceptance of what happens". What an idea! It's a sharp contrast from a Western sensibility; we tend to wait for external things to bring us happiness and contentment. We wait to get married, buy a home, or succeed in our careers, with the understanding that then we will be happy, then we will be content. Yoga asks more of us. *Santosa* is not just a state of mind; it is an action. Contentment is something you practice rather than wait for. We are meant to accept what is, and be joyful in it. No matter what kind of day (or life!) we are having.

Tapas, which literally means 'heat', follows *santosa*. Tapas also carries the meaning of discipline. For most of us, this means our hatha yoga practice, and maybe integrating the *yamas* and *niyamas* off the mat. Discipline means we are dedicated to our practice. It's an important attitude of mind that helps us conquer sloth, or the *tamasic* qualities of our natures. It's a truth in many areas of life that you get out of something what you put into it. Dedication to the practice is what leads us along the path. *Tapas* also works with *shaoca*, as *tapas* implies a dedication to practices which keep the body well. It's interesting that *tapas* follows *santosa*. We have *tapas,* which means self-improvement though discipline, following a *niyama* which tells us to accept what is. The two *niyamas* work together. If you try to practice *sirsasana* (headstand) every week without success, as long as you accept your inability to do it happily, you remain in a state of *santosa*. But you don't stop trying; you continue to practice, week after week. That's the *tapas*, or discipline.

The next niyama is *svadhyaya*, or self-study. In a classical sense, this refers to the study of sacred texts, with the implication that the student would use such texts to deepen his or her self-understanding. In modern Yoga *svadhyaya* has also come to mean self-observation. The application *of svadhyaya* to our consciousness has great impact on our daily lives. It is one of the most important steps we take towards wholeness and integration. To study the self implies distance from the self. To observe the fluctuations of our minds, to observe our emotions and reactions, we must drop back into the witness consciousness. This is the part of our mind that exists beyond the stream of consciousness and the ever-present chatter of fluctuating thoughts. It is with *svadhyaya* that we begin one of the most important steps on the Yogic path; we get beyond our habitual reactions to things (*samskaras*) and start acting in each moment. For example, perhaps through *svadhyaya* you notice that you have a jealousy issue in yoga class. Before, when the class would go into a deep forward bend you would do it despite aching hamstrings or an aching back. Through observing your mind, perhaps you notice that you are doing this only because of an ego desire to be 'good at yoga'. Self-observation helps you to have these realizations, and get beyond habit. Now you wait in your forward bend, observe the state of your body in that moment, and act accordingly rather than out of habit. *Svadhyaya* has the power to teach us so much about ourselves. We learn, above all, how our minds habitually react to certain stimuli, and thus we gain the power to transcend habitual reactions and act from the truth in every moment.

The final *niyama* is one that has so much importance. When I teach *yama* and *niyama* in asana class, I sometimes wish to gloss over this one, as it's an awkward idea for many of us. The last *niyama* is *isvara-pranidhana*, 'to lay all your actions at the feet of God". Often it's translated as simply, surrender. *Isvara* is a Sanskrit word meaning the divine, in a very nondenominational sense. Iyengar writes of *isvara-pranidhana*, "It is offering oneself and all one's actions, however trivial, from cooking a meal to lighting a candle, to the Universal Divine." We could spend a lifetime working just on this *niyama*. *Isvara-pranidhana* speaks especially to one of the five *kleshas* (obstacles) to our happiness; *asmita*, or self-centeredness. To be in a state of surrender means to accept that we are not the center of the universe. We are not the reason for its being, it doesn't revolve around our wants and desires, no matter what our ego says. Many of us yogis think we have transcended ego, at least in some part. But every time you rage at a traffic jam, as if it was put there just to irritate you, you are acting as if you were the center of it all. We can observe this *niyama* by engaging in meditation and *bhakti* (devotional) yoga. When we are in a state of surrender certain things are easier. We know that what happens to us is the work of something greater than ourselves. *Isvara-pranidhana* can also lead us deeper into the heart of gratitude. As we surrender to something higher than ourselves, it becomes easier to be thankful for what we have as a gift from the divine.

Ahhh, Asana

We come to the third limb of the eight-limbed path, asana. For most of us, this is the limb we hold dearest to our hearts. Literally translated, asana means seat or posture. Only two of Patanjali's Yoga Sutras refer to asana; the essence of his teaching is that our posture should be both steady and comfortable. The *Bhagavad Gita* does not instruct regarding hatha Yoga at all. However, there are other ancient texts (such as the *Hatha Yoga Pradikapa)* that do describe the physical discipline of Yoga. Undoubtedly, the physical aspects of Yoga arose later than the philosophical aspects. *Surya namaskar,* which may have had its origins in the beginning of human civilization as a daily devotional offering to the sun, probably became linked to the philosophical teachings of Yoga later. There are different theories regarding the origination of Yoga asanas. Many yogis believe that the poses came to the minds of meditators, who were compelled to rise from their seats and move their bodies into particular positions in order to get energy moving in particular ways. I have also read that many of the asanas come from an ancient Indian system of martial arts, which one can see in postures such as the *Virabhadrasanas.* Whatever the origins of Hatha Yoga, it has become the Yoga most people think of when they think of Yoga.

Why practice asana? Those of us already practicing know that practicing Yoga makes us stronger, more flexible, healthier, and happier. Old injuries or other aches and pains tend to dissipate. The stress response, cause of so much ill health, is decreased. We know that Yoga, on the merits of its physical benefits alone, is a worthwhile endeavor. But there is so much more to it than that.

A traditional view of asana is that it is preparation for meditation, or more specifically, to prepare the body for *padamasana* (lotus pose), which is the classical meditation seat. Prana, or life energy, cannot travel through the body if the energy channels are blocked; thus they must first be unblocked by asana for energy to flow properly and meditation to occur. On a practical level, most of us are not able to sit comfortably for meditation without the opening that comes from Yoga asana practice. Not only do the asanas prepare us physically for meditation, they prepare our minds. By narrowing our mental focus to the practice, we begin to learn *pratyahara* (withdrawal of the senses from that which feeds them). We learn to tune out and disregard stimuli that are unconnected to what we are doing, such as sounds from adjacent rooms. Through asana we also begin to practice *dharana* (concentration), which is another integral step toward meditation. We learn to rein in our wandering minds. Instead of following streams of consciousness, we focus on our breath, or on alignment points and the sensations in our bodies. We are engaged in mental practice just as much as physical.

Hatha Yoga is not just a step on the way to meditation. On its own it can lead us toward enlightenment and integration, with the body as its tool. One of the most important facets of asana practice comes from the word Yoga itself. The root word is "yug" meaning to yoke together. Through Yoga we reconnect body, mind, and spirit. Western thought has for thousands of years acculturated us with a split between mind and body. And most of us behave, and even speak, as if our minds and our bodies were separate entities. Through practice we begin to change this. The attention we pay to our breath becomes a bridge between mind and body. As we practice we begin to reconnect to our bodies. We become aware of our posture, or we begin to crave different, healthier foods. We feel sensations in places in the body that we weren't even aware of. We notice when we're holding our breath because of stress. With awareness comes change.

Another way asana leads us towards wholeness is through the clearing of old energy blockages. All we have ever experienced is held in the body. Thus as we unwind the body we are able to release old injuries as well as unprocessed emotions. Yogic energy anatomy describes energy channels, *nadis*, and energy centers, *chakras*. As the process of asana clears old stuff away, energy begins to flow more easily. Combined with the Yogic practice of *svadhyaya* (self-study) the unconscious begins to becomes conscious. We move past habituated patterns of action and reaction, and are able to act in a more honest and present way.

The mat becomes a microcosm for our lives; and we can bring all of the limbs of Yoga onto the mat and into our practice. We can begin to embrace the *yamas* and the *niyamas* by bringing them into our Yoga practice. We cultivate the skills that we need for meditation. We learn how to truly relax. Asana is a path without end; we can always travel farther, and never run out of things to learn.

"The body is my temple, and asana is my prayer." BKS Iyengar

Breath of Life

So we come to the fourth limb of Patanjali's eight-limbed path of Yoga: *pranayama*. The word *pranayama* is often translated as 'breath control', but it means much more than that. *Pranayama* comes from two Sanskrit words: *prana*, meaning life energy or life force, and *ayama*, meaning extension. So through the practice of working with the breath, we work with our very life energy itself.

The idea of *prana* is one of the most important in all of Yoga. *Prana* is the life energy; it is what differentiates us from that which is not alive. When the life has left our bodies, they are no longer imbued with *prana*. Breath is the main way we sustain our *prana* while alive; thus when we no longer breathe, we die.

Through the practice of Yoga asana, we come to know the breath. We become aware of how we breathe while moving through the postures. In many styles of Yoga, we practice ujjayi pranayama throughout the practice, beginning with this relatively simple way of guiding the breath. Sooner or later, we hopefully begin to carry our breath awareness off the mat. We notice how we breathe (or fail to!) when angered or stressed. Or perhaps we notice that when we are relaxed, out breath is calm and easy. We begin to notice a link between the state of our breath and the state of our mind. Yoga teaches us that *prana* follows consciousness, and that consciousness can be guided by the breath. It's a truth we know instinctively; how many times have you told someone who was upset to "take a deep breath"? We can let our consciousness be guided by the random thoughts, desires, and emotions that arise in the mind, or we can choose to guide our consciousness, by guiding the breath.

There are many types of pranayama practice, differing in both intention and effects. Some are meant to energize, some to relax. For example, the ujjayi pranayama practiced during yoga asana focuses the mind and the will to encourage steadiness and concentration during the practice. Its echoing sound serves as an anchor for a wandering mind. Incorporating *pranayama* into your Yoga practice is a wonderful way to develop concentration and mental clarity. It's an important step on the journey that is Yoga.

Simple pranayama practice for anxiety

Sitting comfortably, allow your breath to settle into a natural pattern. Count the length of a few inhales and exhales. After you have an idea of the length of each, add a 2 count to your exhale. (So if you've been inhaling to an 8, exhaling to 10, make the exhale a 12.) If this length of breath feels comfortable, begin to lengthen the exhale further. Perhaps you can relax enough to allow yourself to find the natural pause that comes after the exhale, before the next inhale begins. The exhalation is a state of surrender and release, relaxing into the flow of life. Finding these qualities in our breath can help us to find them in our lives.

Turning Inward

Now we come to the fifth limb of yoga, *pratyahara*. We can translate this word from the Sanskrit as "to withdraw oneself from that which nourishes the senses". *Pratyahara* comes at an interesting place in our sequence of limbs. It is the last of the *bahirangas*, or external practices which may lead to Yoga. All of the limbs we have looked at so far have a lot to do with the outside world. The yamas and niyamas instruct us on how to behave, and asana and pranayama are both physical practices. Pratyahara is the bridge between these more outward looking practices, and the more inwardly focused limbs which are to come.

What does it mean to 'withdraw our senses'? Well, in our normal daily lives, we are almost constantly under the sway of our senses. The phone rings; we register the sound and jump up. This is how an undisciplined mind works; the senses register an object for perception, and the mind follows. What we seek to do by practicing pratyahara is to sever the automatic link between sensory information coming in followed by mind jumping in response. We seek instead to become so mentally absorbed in something else that our senses don't respond to their normal stimuli. This leads us towards Yoga, or union. We know that when our minds are scattered, constantly jumping here and there, our *prana* (life energy) is also scattered. Many Yogis compare the state of pratyahara to being like a turtle, pulling its limbs and head into its shell.

How do we reach this state of pratyahara? Much like meditation, we cannot 'practice' *pratyahara*. We can only create the situation in which pratyahara can occur. As hatha Yogis, we have tools already available. Through the practice of asana and *pranayama*, we begin to practice sense withdrawal. While practicing asana, we withdraw our senses from all that which is not of the body. We narrow our mental focus to the sensations in our body and to the sound of the breath. We've all been in Yoga classes when sounds from outside intrude upon our practice. When we are not in a state of *pratyahara*, our minds tend to jump at the interruption. Immediately our focus goes from our practice to the noise from outside. Our mind, happy as always to go off on tangents, starts to react. "Oh, how rude those people are to be talking outside of class. How inconsiderate. I never do that when I'm out there..." If instead we are in a state of *pratyahara*, the reaction is different. Perhaps we still register the sound of loud voices from outside, but instead of reacting, we simply go back to paying attention to the breath.

The second of Patanjali's Yoga Sutras states that "Yoga is the cessation of the fluctuations of the mind". Pratyahara, the fifth limb of Yoga, is an important step on the journey to a quiet mind. As we react less and less to the stimuli from outside, we move closer and closer to finding the space between our thoughts. Try setting the stage for *pratyahara* at home. Sit in a comfortable position for a few moments of quiet. Don't seal yourself off from the outside world. Leave the windows open, the phone ringer on. Bring your attention to your breath, or say a mantra silently to yourself. Let the sounds and smells from outside wash over you. Let any internal urge to move, or scratch an itch, fade away. See if you can be non-reactive; let input from your senses just be background, as your mind quiets and stills.

Unity from Diversity

The sixth limb of Yoga, *dharana*, means concentration. With this limb we have come to the first of the *antaranga*, or internal limbs of Yoga. All of the other limbs have been intrinsically involved with how we relate to the outside world, whether by teaching us moral precepts for our life in society, or by learning to tune out that outside world through *pratyahara*. This limb, and the ones that follow, get down to the nitty-gritty; the calming of the mind, and the finding of the state of Yoga.

So what is concentration? Many classical yogis define it as 12 seconds of unbroken attention. That may seem like no big deal, until you try it. For most of us, our minds are constantly awash with waves of thought (*vrittis*). The Yoga Sutras of Patanjali describe three main types of *vrittis*. (And I have to say, I don't think modern psychology could explain it any better.) One grouping is the thoughts and mental images that arise from sensory stimuli. Thus we can see how our previous limb, *pratyahara* (withdrawal of the senses from that which stimulates them) helps to prepare us for these later stages. Another type of *vrtti* is memory; the mental images and thoughts that arise from our pasts. The final type of *vrtti* is that which comes from anticipation of the future. Take the time to observe your wandering thoughts, and you will see that almost every one falls into one of these three categories. *Dharana*, or concentration, is the opposite of this. Instead of jumping around from thought to thought, image to image, the mind is focused on one object.

There are two main types of classical techniques for practicing *dharana*. The first involves focusing on a place in your energetic body, and directing all of your attention there. The *chakras*, (energy centers), are common foci for this type of *dharana* practice. A second practice would be to focus internally on a mental image, such as a flame, or a mantra or prayer. The important thing is that what you focus on is a single thing; the point is to take the many streams of our thoughts and direct them to one object of concentration. For example, if your object of concentration is an image of a flame, the unbidden *vrttis* would fade away in the face of a conscious *vrtti*; "flame, flame, flame." Any time your concentration wavered, you would bring your mind back to the image of the flame.

One of the most wonderful things about the limbs is the way they work together. We can see how the previous limbs have laid the groundwork for this work in concentration. When we practice asana, we are learning to concentrate. All of our attention is internal. One of the reasons teachers give alignment instructions is to give yogis a place to direct their minds, as well as to deepen the physical practice. We also prepare for *dharana* by our yogic practice of *dhrishti* (gaze). By keeping our gaze focused, the mind follows. If we also work with *pranayama*, we have narrowed our focus of attention even further, to the breath.

You can start to integrate *dharana* more thoroughly into your asana practice. Rather than letting your attention flit from body part to body part, from your breath to the music to the sound of the teacher's voice, choose one focus of attention for one particular practice. A good choice would be breath, to be more specific, a particular quality of your breath such as its sound or its depth. Another interesting choice would be a body part; for example, the toe of your right foot. Can you keep your attention there for a few moments? If your mind wanders, can you remember to bring it back?

As your mind strengthens, and your ability to concentrate increases, your mind becomes more able to calm itself. Rather than constantly fluctuating, it can be easily brought back to a state of wholeness. Which is, after all, the goal of Yoga.

Journey to the Center

Now that we've learned to concentrate, we move on to the seventh limb of yoga: *dhyana*. *Dhyana* is meditation. First we should be clear about what meditation is not. Meditation is not relaxation, although you must be relaxed to meditate. Meditation is not being led through a guided visualization, although such practices have great merit. Meditation, in the classical, Yogic, sense, is the stilling of the movements of the mind. This is a fairly simple statement, but there is a great deal that comes from that quiet mind.

As with *pratyahara*, our practice is to set the stage to allow meditation to happen. The earlier limbs have certainly done their part in preparation. B.K.S. Iyengar writes in Light on Life, "You cannot meditate from a starting point of stress or bodily infirmity." The earlier limbs have certainly done their part in preparation. Through asana, *pranayama*, and other Yogic practices, we have prepared our bodies to sit in meditation, and our minds to begin to calm. For some of us, our yoga asana practice has become a form of meditation. We are able to withdraw our senses, concentrate on an aspect of the practice, and find a quiet mind for stretches of time during the practice.

It can be difficult to delineate these final three limbs of yoga. They are *samyama*, the Yoga of final integration. It can be hard to differentiate where one ends and the next begins. In the state of *dharana*, we have created a link between our mind and the object of our concentration, and begun to maintain that link. *Dharana* becomes *dhyana* when the flow is continuous, and our attention does not waver. Classical Yoga states that *dharana* is reached when the attention is focused for 12 seconds. It becomes *dhyana*, or meditation, when the flow has been sustained for 144 seconds. It certainly doesn't seem that long, unless you're the one trying to do it. *Dharana* sets the stage for meditation to happen by allowing the *vrttis* (fluctuations of the mind) to slow.

How do you know that you are meditating? The effort to sustain your attention disappears. In *dharana* there is still the implication that you are trying to focus your attention on something. To go back to the example of one concentrating on the mental image of a flame, in *dharana* you are still working to keep that internal focus on the flame. You may still be aware of *vrttis* (thought-waves) struggling to arise in the background of your mind. Once you have segued into meditation, that sensation of trying to concentrate is gone. You are simply concentrating, absorbed in the object of the meditation. You are now in a relationship with the object of your meditation. And so you remain, until the first *vrtti* pops us. "Wow! I'm meditating!"

Meditation is not trying to make your mind blank. Who would want a completely empty mind? Rather, your mind is alive with potential. Without tons of thoughts and memories and anticipations of the future crowding in, you have a chance to see what you actually are. This is why, from that brief Yoga sutra, "Yoga is the cessation of the fluctuations of the mind," one could elaborate the whole philosophy of Yoga. For when we have reached the state of meditation, our ego has dropped away enough for us to merge with the object of the meditation. We are gifted with clarity. We begin to see and feel our true nature, and that nature of all that is. We have begun to feel our *union*, our oneness, with everything else that is. In this state, we begin to see what we truly are. In the words of B.K.S. Iyengar, "It is bringing the turbulent sea to a state of flat clam. This calm is not torpid or inert. It is a deep tranquility, pregnant with all the potential of creation."

Who am I?

If someone asks me, "Who are you?", I can answer fairly easily. I am a mother. I am a wife, a yoga student and teacher, a writer. I could list things that I am for hours, as all of us could. "Who am I?" is the fundamental question of Yoga practice. We use many different ways to answer it. However, according to Yogic thought, all of the answers that I supplied can only lead to unhappiness. This is because they are answers based on my status in the material world (*prakriti.*) As such, these ideas I hold about myself can only lead to loss. The world is constantly in flux. If we base our happiness and our joy on characteristics of our lives in the world, we will be disappointed. If my happiness comes from identifying as a Yoga teacher, what happens if I can no longer teach Yoga? Through the practice of Yoga, we strip away all that is of the ego, to get at the root of what we truly are.

That is what happens when we experience the eighth limb of Yoga, *samadhi*. Sometimes it is translated as bliss; you could also call it a state of pure spiritual absorption. You could even call it enlightenment. When one is able to stay in meditation for a sustained amount of time, one might reach *samadhi*. According to classical Yogis, if one stays in a state of *dhyana* (meditation) for 1,728 seconds (12 times 12 times 12), one enters the first stage of *samadhi*. *Samadhi* is no less than the union with the divine Self that lives in all of us.

When considering both *dharana* and *dhyana*, we have used the terms subject and object. In *dharana*, the subject (you) has created a link with the object of your thoughts, through concentration. When this sustained concentration has become *dhyana*, meditation, it is said that there is then a relationship between subject and object. To go back to the example of the flame, once we have reached samadhi, there is no more "I" watching the flame, and there is no more flame. Each has dissolved into the other. There is no more subject and no more object. The illusory boundaries which separate us from all that is not us have dissolved, and we are at one.

In the state of samadhi, "I" disappears. The identification of self with the ego fades away, and one knows that one is truly Self. The *samskaras* (mental disturbances) are gone, and we are able to see all things with clarity. *Samadhi* fades; it is an experience, and it passes. However, some yogis will eventually remain in a continuous state of samadhi, in this unbridled clarity. This is called *kaivalya*. Those who dwell in this state live in the world, but they are not of it. They are not subject to the world's vicissitudes, as they dwell in their Self.

According to Yogic thought, union with something greater than ourselves is what we all seek, although we may not know it. Most people spend their lives looking for bliss, or happiness, or a sense of connection. Many of these paths are destructive; just look at those who seek union by using drugs, alcohol, other people, or risky behavior. Other paths are not so destructive to the naked eye; look to those who spend their lives questing after more and more money. Yet inside there is that same soul yearning for union.

When we find samadhi, we also find the answer to the question, "Who am I?" The answer, of course, is "I am that. That is God."

978-0-595-41740-
0-595-41740-X

Made in United States
North Haven, CT
08 November 2022

26417163R00048